MANAGING WEIGHT

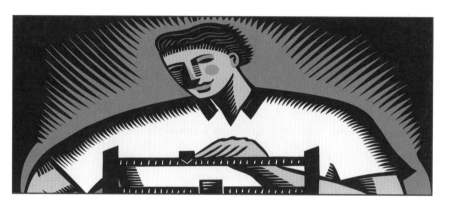

A PRACTICAL HANDBOOK TO PROGRAM PLANNING

50 GREAT IDEAS FOR WORKING WELL

Wellness Councils of America
9802 Nicholas Street, Suite 315, Omaha, NE 68114
Phone: (402) 827-3590   Fax: (402) 827-3594

www.welcoa.org

COPYRIGHT AND DISCLOSURE

Managing Weight
A Practical Handbook to Program Planning
50 Great Ideas for Working Well

EXECUTIVE EDITOR
David M. Hunnicutt, PhD
President, Wellness Councils of America

ASSISTANT EDITOR
Brittanie Leffelman
Assistant to the President, Wellness Councils of America

AUTHORS
Craig Johnson, Carie Maguire, Sara Spurgin, Marice Reyes
Writing Staff, Wellness Councils of America

DESIGN
David Trouba
Creative Director, Wellness Councils of America

PUBLISHED AND DISTRIBUTED BY
The Wellness Councils of America (WELCOA)
9802 Nicholas Street, Suite 315
Omaha, NE 68114-2106

Phone: (402) 827-3590
Fax: (402) 827-3594

WEBSITE: www.welcoa.org
E-MAIL: wellworkplace@welcoa.org

© 2001 Wellness Councils of America

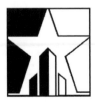

TABLE OF CONTENTS

PREFACE

For over a decade, The Wellness Councils of America (WELCOA) has been dedicated to building and sustaining world-class corporate wellness programs. Our staff, directors, medical advisors, and local councils have assisted hundreds of organizations in transforming their corporate cultures into health conscious, wellness-oriented environments. With over 2,000 member organizations throughout North America and 11 locally affiliated community "Wellness Councils," WELCOA is recognized as the premier resource for worksite wellness.

In our continuing efforts to build successful wellness initiatives, we are proud to introduce a new series of books titled *50 Great Ideas for Working Well.* Each book focuses on a specific health concern and provides 50 tips on how to implement programs on each topic. Many of these "in the trenches" ideas have been drawn from companies we have worked with in our continuous effort to build "well worksites."

In this book, we have provided additional information for you to utilize in the development of your programs. Much of this information comes in the form of online technology—a fast and convenient way for you to get started. However, with the pace of today's technology, websites can change overnight. If this does occur, don't let it end your search, there are plenty of other options out there.

Keep in mind that these 50 great ideas are by no means an exhaustive list—these tips are meant to stimulate critical thinking and generate new ideas for your own wellness initiatives. In addition, we encourage you to send us your ideas and communicate your own successful wellness efforts.

Lastly, we would like to give a special thanks to the practitioners who have contributed to these 50 great ideas. We hope that their creativity and hard work will inspire your own efforts in creating a well workplace.

"People may doubt what you say,
but they will believe what you do."
—Lewis Cass

WEIGHT MANAGEMENT AT A GLANCE...

✓ Obesity kills. Our nation's top three causes of death—heart disease, cancer, and stroke—are directly related to an overweight and obese population.[1]

✓ Each year, more than 300,000 people, many of whom work in American businesses, will die because of issues related to obesity and physical inactivity. [2]

✓ Health care expenditures due to obesity and physical inactivity equal an estimated $12.7 billion, including $2.6 billion as a result of mild obesity and $10.1 billion due to moderate to severe obesity.[3]

✓ When all is said and done, the direct and indirect costs of obesity are estimated to be in excess of $100 billion per year.[4]

✓ In 1998, promotion costs for popular candy bars were $10 to $50 million, up to $115 million for soft drinks, and just over a billion dollars for the McDonald's restaurant chain. Conversely, The National Cancer Institute annually invests $1 million in its campaign to promote fruits and vegetables.[5]

"No diet will remove all the fat from your body because the brain is entirely fat. Without a brain you might look good, but all you could do is run for public office."

—Covert Bailey
(fitness expert)

OBESITY...IT'S ALL AROUND US

or years, an overweight workforce was of little concern to the nation's employers. But with the dramatic increase in the number of people who are now overweight and/or obese, as well as better information quantifying both the direct and indirect costs associated with this insidious health concern, employers of all sizes are now taking notice.

In a study of over 3,000 employees of First Chicago Bank, employees who were at least 20% over ideal weight had health care costs (based on medical claims) 50% greater than employees of normal weight.[6] Additionally, in a study of over 17,000 members of an HMO, those with a Body Mass Index (BMI) of 35 kg/m² used more medication and had 2 times the medication costs of non-obese people (BMI 20-25 kg/m²). [7]

Think your company's not affected? Think again.

Statistically, if there are 100 people in your company or department...[8]	
1	uses cocaine
50	feel they're under moderate stress
10	are heavy drinkers
30	smoke
60	**sit all day to do their work**
27	**have cardiovascular disease**
10	**have high blood pressure**
5	**have diagnosed diabetes**
5	**have undiagnosed diabetes**
25	**or more have high blood cholesterol**
35	**are overweight by 20% or more**
50	don't wear their safety belts regularly
7	use marijuana

Promoting weight management in the workplace is not easy, but it can be done. When construction manufacturer Caterpillar saw medical expenses increasing at double-digit rates in the early 1990s, they took notice. When healthcare costs were projected to exceed $1 billion in the years to come, they took action. Caterpillar got aggressive and created the Healthy Balance℠ Program.[9]

After identifying overweight as their #1 preventable health risk, Caterpillar took the appropriate steps by providing healthy foods in cafeterias and vending machines, holding on-site exercise classes, and giving reimbursements for fitness clubs. At the start of the program, more than 60% of eligible participants were classified overweight with a BMI greater than 25. Since implementation, 4,700 employees have lost weight, and medical expenses have lowered for program participants compared to non-participants. Savings in medical expenses are anticipated to surpass $700 million by 2015, showing that shedding the pounds can pack on the savings.[9]

High Dollar Loss!

In lieu of sound strategies, Americans have repeatedly shown a willful suspension of disbelief for get-thin-quick products. Check out the statistics below.

✓ Consumers spend $33 billion a year on the diet industry.[10]

✓ Americans spend $40 million a year on gut-busters.[11]

✓ Every year, about 8 million Americans sign up for weight loss programs that offer a quick and easy fix.[12]

✓ An estimated $6 billion a year is spent on fraudulent diet products.[13]

"From a standpoint of promoting good health and preventing disease, weight is a major factor...all companies want healthy employees. Therefore, it makes sense for companies to try to help employees achieve desirable weights."

—Dr. Don Gemson
Medical Director, Merrill Lynch

3

50
Great Ideas
For Managing Weight

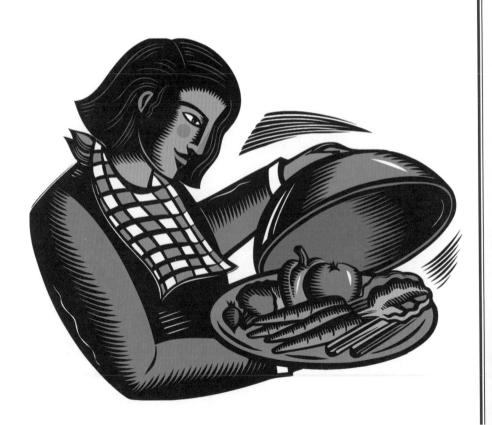

Great Idea #1

Walk out on your job! A walking program is one of the best ways to get lots of employees moving. The entire business community of Kearney, NE, holds a "walk out on your job" fitness extravaganza once a year—a great start to worksite physical activity.

Take Action!

**Organize an annual company walk.
Not only will this raise awareness, but it will also get your company moving from top to bottom.**

Great Idea #2

When it's time to change, you've got to rearrange. Start by changing the contents of your vending machines. You don't have to do anything too drastic, but consider this: By simply substituting one cup of plain unbuttered popcorn for a one-ounce bag of potato chips, you save 120 calories and 8.5 grams of fat![14] Inform your employees of the "good" and "bad" food found in vending machines. Remember, it's impossible to eat healthy if you don't know what's in the snack. If you're still hungry to do more, how about moving the entire machine? Find a spot that takes a good walk to get to—this will help burn off some of the calories they consume in the process.

Take Action!

Get in touch with the contents and caloric values of the foods in your vending machines. Once you've listed them out, post the information on the vending machine itself. And while all this is going on, start looking for vendors who can provide healthy snacks that you can place along side the traditional favorites of chips and candy.

GREAT IDEA #3

how them the menu. Eating out doesn't have to be unhealthy. Inform employees how to make healthy choices and avoid high-fat, high-calorie meals when they're dining out. At one fast food establishment, a bacon cheeseburger averages 420 more calories than a plain burger[14]—that's valuable info for your employees. Also highlight menu items that can be deceiving. Sautéed foods, for example, are pan fried in butter. And although we generally think of salads as being healthy, chef and Caesar salads contain a number of high-fat, high-calorie ingredients.

TAKE ACTION!

Start a collection of menus from local eateries and identify the best options for your employees. Hold a class to get the word out.

Vending machines are a $36 billion a year business. While soda remains most popular, Snickers candy bars are the favorite snack.[15]

6

GREAT IDEA #4

Data is what matta'. Determining employees' interests is vital to designing an intervention that works. You need to know what you're working with before you can know where to start. Begin by gathering employee health data—you can then use this information to develop a database and properly address weight management. As the largest insurer in West Virginia, Public Employees Insurance Association (PEIA) collects and cross-references employee health data in a comprehensive database and has been able to use the data to target risk factors and reduce health care costs. Without this database, PEIA would be unable to reach its primary audience and thus unable to modify behaviors.

TAKE ACTION!

Design a survey to assess your employees' interests. If you're not the surveying type, then schedule face-to-face conversations or interviews with employees throughout your organization—and ask them the hard questions about their desires to lose weight.

GREAT IDEA #5

Offer competitions galore. A number of innovative companies have enlisted large groups of employees in competitions to lose weight. By engaging teams of employees in physical activity and healthier eating, individuals are able to lose weight with the backing of the organization. It is important to note that the results of each team's progress are measured collectively—using large industrial scales. Not only does this approach ensure anonymity, but it also provides unparalleled peer support.

TAKE ACTION!

Order an incentive campaign today. There are dozens of incentive campaigns that encourage employees to compete in healthy ways toward their goals. For great incentive campaigns, check out those offered by Health Enhancement Solutions at www.hesonline.com.

> *"You could get mauled by a bear and die. You could fall off a cliff and die. You could get shot by a hunter and die. Or, you could stay home on the couch, eat potato chips and die."*
>
> **— John Naisbitt,
> High Tech High Touch**

GREAT IDEA # 6

ook to the top. There's no question that programs with active senior level support are the ones most likely to succeed. Your senior level executives should serve as an example for the rest of the company to follow. Not only did Fortis Health, formerly John Alden Life Insurance, in Miami, Florida find this idea beneficial through their senior level "boot camp," they also found it helpful in their efforts to create a more supportive environment for all employees.

TAKE ACTION!

Get your senior level people involved by offering executive level health promotion programs. A great way to do this is through health screenings. We suggest you check out HealthScreen America at www.healthscreenamerica.com and inquire about their executive screening program.

GREAT IDEA #7

eam up. Secure a wellness team comprised of employees at different fitness levels. While a person in top shape will know what works well for people in the same category, he or she might not know how to reach those that don't exercise at all. Having multiple perspectives can expand your program participation base.

TAKE ACTION!

Invite individuals who are struggling with weight management issues to become part of your health promotion team—and listen, listen, listen.

GREAT IDEA #8

Back to school. Educate employees on diet and physical activity. This can be in the form of seminars, pamphlets, brochures, and other informative material. Townsend Engineering is excelling in this critical programming area. Located in Des Moines, IA, this equipment manufacturer offers on-going lunch-n-learn sessions on subjects such as nutrition, cholesterol, and cooking.

TAKE ACTION!

Contact all of the major organizations that provide health information. From WELCOA to Vitality to Personal Best, these organizations have answers to the health information dilemma. Struggling with budgetary issues? Don't overlook your local community health agencies and hospitals.

In 1995, the total economic cost of obesity in the U.S. was estimated to be nearly $100 billion.[16]

GREAT IDEA #9

Keep employees in the know. Provide information on exercise guidelines. Most Americans report using diet, physical activity, or both for weight loss—but only a minority uses the recommended combination.[10] The Surgeon General recommends 30 minutes of moderate physical activity on most days of the week.[17]

TAKE ACTION!

Order your copy of the *Surgeon General's Report on Physical Activity*. You can obtain it by contacting the Centers for Disease Control and Prevention in Atlanta.

GREAT IDEA #10

Family matters. When employees aren't at work, they're usually with their families. And, family members tend to live similar lifestyles—so if you don't exercise, your children will most likely not exercise either. *The Journal of the American Medical Association* revealed that the risk factors children have will become chronic diseases as adults.[18]

TAKE ACTION!

Make your programs available and convenient to all family members—including children. There's no question that it takes more effort on your part to do this, but the results will be far better than if you ask employees to go it alone.

An estimated 13% of children ages 6 to 11 are overweight.[19]

An estimated 14% of adolescents ages 12 to 19 are overweight.[19]

GREAT IDEA #11

Get connected. Providing daily health tips via e-mail is a fast and easy way to get the word out on weight management. Fortune 500 giant Union Pacific Railroad distributes an electronic newsletter to employees via the company's Intranet. Known as the "Healthy Hound Tip O' the Day," this daily electronic message is consistently rated as the most popular segment of UPRR's online health newsletter.

TAKE ACTION!

Check out Mayo Clinic's website at www.mayohealth.org. It's a great site for information customized to your own personal needs.

GREAT IDEA #12

Take it to the tube. Provide healthy messages on screen savers and network televisions. Charleston Area Medical Center in West Virginia employs some 5,000 people at three separate facilities. In order to get their health messages out, they broadcast wellness programs in staff lounges on their 24-hour hospital television station.

TAKE ACTION!

Get in touch with WinningHabits.com—a web-based wellness application service provider. They can customize wellness web pages for organizations to provide health information for employees. Log on to www.winninghabits.com or call 1-800-454-4598 to find out what works best for your company.

GREAT IDEA #13

Dispel the myths about fad diets. No matter which fad diet is considered, the strategies are typically the same—unusual combinations and unrealistic expectations. But day after day, Americans are routinely duped. In fact, Americans spend an estimated $6 billion a year on fraudulent diet products.[14] By educating employees on the right way to lose weight, the chances of success are exponentially increased.

TAKE ACTION!

To help dispel the myths about fad diets, check out www.americanheart.org/Heart_and_Stroke_A_Z_Guide/fad.html and download their publication that zeroes in on the war against fad diets.

Consumers spend $33 billion annually for weight loss products and services.[10]

GREAT IDEA #14

Note teachable moments. There are times when employees are naturally more interested in maintaining and/or improving their health. Birthdays and pregnancies are just two prime examples. During these times, employees are naturally more contemplative—and thus more receptive to important health messages. Be in tune with important events in employees' lives and use these events to promote a healthier lifestyle.

TAKE ACTION!

If you're interested in learning more on how to help people change for the better, then check out Dr. James Prochaska's book, *Changing for Good*. The book is available at most bookstores—ISBN # is 0-380-72572-X—and retails for $12.00.

GREAT IDEA #15

Get creative. It has been estimated that most Americans watch about four hours of television per day, or twenty-eight hours per week.[20] Let's face it, people aren't going to entirely give up their TV. To get some people moving, you're going to have to get creative. Provide exercises that they can do while watching TV or working at a computer, such as shoulder shrugs, crunches, jumping jacks, and stretching.

TAKE ACTION!

Provide your employees with brief one-page handouts on simple strengthening and stretching exercises. These exercises are routinely available through most publications like *Runner's World* and *Walking* magazines.

A TV Guide poll showed that 23% of those surveyed would give up their TV viewing habits for $25,000, and 46% would only settle for a million dollars. Conversely, a million dollars still wasn't enough for 25% of those polled.[21]

GREAT IDEA #16

Combine high-tech with high-touch. Utilize Internet technology to deliver a behavioral weight loss program. This can be an effective channel of communication and support. A study from *The Journal of the American Medical Association* indicated that a group who received interactive behavioral lessons and feedback from a therapist via e-mail lost more weight than those who were denied online interaction.[22]

TAKE ACTION!

Contact Health Media Inc. and inquire about their tailored health behavior solutions. For an overview of the products and services they offer, check out their website at www.healthmedia.com.

GREAT IDEA #17

Make the first move. Yogi Berra once said, "If people don't want to come out to the park, nobody's going to stop 'em." Miami Valley Hospital, an employer of 5,000 people located in Dayton, OH, has taken this message to heart. Instead of waiting for their employees to get involved, health promoters personally deliver information on specific health issues and corporate programs to every unit of the hospital.

TAKE ACTION!

Contact your organization's health care provider and research what it would take to get a health fair set up at your location. Not only are they great fun, but they're extremely informative as well.

GREAT IDEA #18

e colorful.** By implementing a red, yellow, and green light system nutritional choices can be improved in the company cafeteria. Foods marked with a red light are high in fat and calories, while green light foods indicate healthy choices. In addition, provide general nutrition guidelines on big posters that can easily be seen.

TAKE ACTION!

An excellent source for nutrition information is the American Dietetic Association. Check them out at www.eatright.org.

"Let me put it this way. According to my girth, I should be a 90-foot redwood."
—Erma Bombeck

GREAT IDEA #19

A lotta' agua. Americans consume an average of 54.5 gallons of soft drinks on an annual basis—much of it out of habit.[24] This results in excess and unnecessary calorie consumption. Instead of having a soda break, encourage employees to substitute water. Consider placing water coolers throughout the building so that water is easily accessible. You may also want to limit the number of soda machines to discourage soda breaks. Continental Western Group holds an annual water campaign called "Make Mine Water." This year's goal was 30,000 ounces and the 160 employees were able to reach the mark in just three weeks.

TAKE ACTION!

Explore what it would cost to have bottled water placed in the vending machines, or better yet, contract with a company to provide water coolers throughout your organization.

GREAT IDEA #20

P romote BMI. Body Mass Index (BMI) is calculated by dividing weight in kilograms by height in meters squared. A BMI of 25.0 to 29.9 kg/m^2 is considered overweight and 30 kg/m^2 and above is considered obese. Posting simple BMI charts at key locations throughout the organization can raise awareness.

TAKE ACTION!

**To view a BMI table, visit the
National Heart Lung and Blood Institute online at
www.nhlbi.nih.gov/guidelines/obesity/bmi_tbl.htm.**

"Top 10 Signs You've Eaten Too Much"

10. *Hundreds of volunteers have started to stack sandbags around you.*

9. *You are responsible for a slight but measurable shift in the Earth's axis.*

8. *Doctor tells you your weight would be perfect for a man 17 feet tall.*

7. *Every escalator you step on immediately grinds to a halt.*

6. *Worlds fattest man sends you a telegram warning you to "back off!"*

5. *A button blows off your 501 jeans and kills a guy.*

4. *People leaving a showing of Free Willy tell you "you were great!"*

3. *Getting off your couch requires help from the fire department.*

2. *It's several generations before your region recovers from the shortage of dinner rolls.*

1. *Your ears are oozing creamed corn.*

—David Letterman's Book of Top Ten Lists and Zesty Lo-Cal Chicken Recipes[23]

GREAT IDEA #21

Use the great pyramid. Provide employees with tools that can help them understand what and how much should be included in their diet. This will raise their awareness of the food groups and their recommended number of servings. Remember, most people want to eat healthy, but often don't know what's included in a healthy diet.

TAKE ACTION!

The United States Department of Agriculture has an interactive food guide pyramid that can help get you started. Check it out at www.usda.gov.

GREAT IDEA #22

Become a stair master. Encourage employees to take the stairs. Several worksites have found that people who began using the stairs improved their overall fitness by 10 to 15%. Promoting stair use may be easier than you think. One study found that a sign encouraging employees to take the stairs increased stair use from 5 to 14%.[25]

TAKE ACTION!

Identify every stairwell in your organization and make sure that the doors remain open and that they are accessible. Also, make sure to post signs that encourage people to use 'em!

GREAT IDEA #23

Get cookin'. Encourage employees to plan their meals ahead of time so they don't fall victim to fast food meals or takeout dinners. Unlike the days our mothers cooked from scratch, three-quarters of Americans don't know at 4:00 pm what they are going to eat for dinner that evening.[26] To help employees plan ahead, provide meal cards that contain healthy recipes. Employees can then plan their meals for the week and know ahead of time what they need to get from the store.

TAKE ACTION!

Check out a great cookbook—*The Cooking Cardiologist: Recipes to Help Lower Cholesterol, Reduce Risk of Heart Disease, Control Weight, Increase Vitality and Longevity* **by Dr. Richard Collins. Look for it in your local bookstores—the ISBN# is: 1889462055.**

Americans spend over $1 billion a day in restaurants or takeout.[27]

In 2000, Americans spent $110 billion on fast food alone. That's more than we spent on movies, books, magazines, newspapers, videos, and recorded music—combined.[28]

Great Idea #24

If you build it they will come. There's more than one way to carry out a weight loss initiative. Use what's available to you to promote a healthy lifestyle with your employees. Whether it involves putting exercise equipment in offices or simply providing pamphlets on healthy eating, using all available resources will further ensure the success of your program. Union Pacific Railroad has taken progressive measures to combat the spread of obesity among its 56,000 employees. Creativity counts, and by converting railcars into fitness facilities, UPRR has taken good health on the road.

Take Action!

Step back and take a hard look at the core business of your company and when, where, and how people consume calories. From here, identify the five most important things that can be done to help your employees eat in healthier ways.

Great Idea #25

Shop 'til you drop...the pounds. Provide skills training for shopping in grocery stores. The odd number of aisles, the "hidden foods," and the mazelike structure all testify that grocery store design has a psychology similar to casinos—stay longer and spend more. By informing your employees about the design and layout of grocery stores, as well as providing them with smart shopping tips, your efforts will greatly assist employees in avoiding unnecessary, and perhaps even unhealthy purchases.

Take Action!

Contact a local dietitian who can provide seminars on how to successfully shop in grocery stores. If you do it right, these seminars will be packed!

The average person in the West eats 50 tons of food and drinks 11,000 gallons of liquid during his or her lifetime.[29]

GREAT IDEA #26

Recognize extreme measures. Just because someone is not overweight doesn't necessarily mean that they're healthy. Some people are so obsessed with the "perfect" body that they'll do anything to attain it. Eating disorders such as bulimia and anorexia nervosa are serious conditions—mortality rates are as high as 20%.[30]

TAKE ACTION!

Get familiar with the warning signs of these disorders, and at the very least post some informational posters that include a number or hotline for help. The National Association of Anorexia Nervosa and Associated Disorders has a national hotline—1-847-831-3438.

GREAT IDEA #27

The mind matters. Offer self-esteem programs along with your weight management programs. One in four people who see a primary care physician about weight problems also has a psychiatric illness—usually depression.[31] In addition, overweight people are likely to share common prejudices about themselves.[30] People with similar lifestyles and behaviors tend to find strength in numbers. A self-esteem component may be just what it takes to keep some program participants from dropping out.

TAKE ACTION!

To learn more about the psychological aspects of health related behaviors, check out a great book by Brian Luke Seaward called, *Health of the Human Spirit: Spiritual Dimensions for Personal Health.* It's available at www.Amazon.com and retails for $26.

GREAT IDEA #28

Read the fine print. Host a course on reading food labels. It's not just fat, but total calories, serving size, protein, carbohydrates, and vitamins and minerals that are essential in maintaining a healthy weight. Sadly, despite their best attempts to eat healthier foods, millions of Americans can't read food labels. Without the necessary skills to decipher food labels, your employees will only be guessing at which foods are healthy and which foods are not.

TAKE ACTION!

Contract with a local dietitian to offer a course in reading food and nutritional labels. Emphasize personal skill building and the ability to consistently pick low-fat and nutritional foods.

Know Your "Fat Words"

Fat-Free:
> *less than 0.5 grams of fat per serving*

Low-Fat:
> *3 grams of fat (or less) per serving*

Lean:
> *Less than 10 grams of fat, 4 grams of saturated fat, and 95 milligrams of cholesterol per serving*

Cholesterol-Free:
> *Less than 2 milligrams of cholesterol and 2 grams (or less) of saturated fat per serving*

> **—Food and Drug Administration**[32]

GREAT IDEA #29

A wolf in sheep's clothing. Some employees might be thin, but this doesn't necessarily mean that they are healthy. A collection of studies has found that a lean population is typically comprised of smokers, those who have lost weight as a result of disease, and those who have maintained a lean weight by balancing physical activity and caloric intake.[33]

TAKE ACTION!

Identify and publicize those individuals who are making the effort to lose weight by incorporating healthy changes and habits into their lifestyle. Make sure it's clear that there are no short cuts, and that smoking as a means of weight loss will not be recognized or rewarded.

GREAT IDEA #30

Bull's-eye! Adapt weight loss programs to meet the needs of specific populations. As with almost all wellness efforts, there is no cookie cutter approach that works for everyone. Different organizations have different populations. From age, gender, and interests to stages of readiness, effective programs require a custom fit approach that takes a population's characteristics into consideration.

TAKE ACTION!

At the beginning of every weight loss class that's offered in your organization, make sure to gather as much information on the participants as possible. In so doing, you'll gain a better understanding of what will be required to help people change.

According to the American Journal of Health Promotion (AJHP), each year U.S. businesses spend a substantial amount of money addressing the following diseases— all of which are related to obesity.[3]

Coronary Heart Disease—$6.4 billion

Hypertension—$3.5 billion

Type II Diabetes—$2.8 billion

Stroke—$2.0 billion

Gallbladder Disease—$1.5 billion

Hypercholesterolemia—$837 million

Endometrial Cancer—$415 million

Osteoarthritis of the Knee—$211 million

GREAT IDEA #31

Be realistic. A reasonable timeline for 10% reduction in body weight is six months of therapy. For overweight patients with BMI's in the typical range of 27-35 kg/m^2, a decrease of 300 to 500 kcal per day will result in weight losses of about one half to one pound a week, and a 10% loss in 10 months.[34] Quicker results aren't necessarily better results. In fact, steady weight loss over time is preferred, and more likely to be sustained.

TAKE ACTION!

Because weight loss is a slow process, it is important to emphasize other forms of positive feedback in addition to the number of pounds lost. For example, small successes like the number of days of consistent adherence to caloric consumption should be rewarded. In addition, things like counting the number of days that included physical activity can be another great way to provide positive feedback.

GREAT IDEA #32

Substitution is not always the solution. While substitutions can be healthier, this is not always the case. For instance, if you substitute a bagel for a doughnut, keep in mind that a bagel is high in carbohydrates, and may be so dense that it's equal to eight slices of bread.

TAKE ACTION!

Arm your employees with calorie counters, or better yet, identify and distribute low-fat, low-calorie menu options from each of your employees' favorite eateries.

Great Idea #33

Make it a combo. The majority of individuals trying to lose weight fail to balance caloric intake and physical activity. *The Journal of the American Medical Association* reported that only 21.5% of men and 19.4% of women reported using the recommended combination of eating fewer calories and engaging in at least 150 minutes of leisure time physical activity per week.[10] Educate employees on the importance of combining both physical activity and a limited caloric intake as a proper means of controlling weight.

Take Action!

To learn more about the art and science of weight management, check out the audiotapes from the American College of Sports Medicine's 47th Annual Meeting. A list of the tapes is available from www.mobiletape.com.

"It [permanent weight loss] is harder than smoking cessation, it's harder than blood pressure control, it's harder than exercise. It's probably the single most difficult risk to manage in a population."

**David Anderson, Ph.D.,
Executive Consultant,
Programs & Technology,
StayWell Health Management**

GREAT IDEA #34

What's up doc? Encourage individuals to get routine medical checkups. *The Journal of the American Medical Association* reports that obese individuals who were advised to lose weight by their physicians or health care providers were three times more likely to report an attempt to reduce their weight than those who did not see a health care professional.[35]

TAKE ACTION!

Create a calendar where twice a year you send out friendly reminders to your employees to think about scheduling their next medical checkup. Not only will this keep preventive measures on the front burner, it will also challenge your employees to think about their health status.

GREAT IDEA #35

Show them the fat! Illustrate the amount of fat in some popular high-fat foods by putting the equivalent amount of Crisco or butter in a jar. For example, a McDonald's Big Mac has 34 grams of fat.[36] Crisco has 12 grams of fat per tablespoon.[37] So you could dish up three tablespoons of Crisco to represent the amount of fat in one Big Mac. This can be quite convincing.

TAKE ACTION!

Create a display in a prominent place within your organization where employees can view how much fat is actually contained in a variety of fast foods. In addition to creating this visual display, it is helpful to create a one-page handout detailing the amount of fat employees would find in their "favorite" foods at all of the major fast food chains.

One hundred thirty-one pound Takeru Kobayashi set a new world record by eating 50 hot dogs in 12 minutes—buns and all! He consumed approximately 19,000 calories and 900 grams of fat—the amount of calories the average American consumes in a week. In addition, he ate almost two weeks' worth of fat.[14]

GREAT IDEA #36

Know the net. It is estimated that by 2005, one billion people will be connected to the Internet.[38] With more and more people now searching for health information, employers would be wise to provide a list of credible sites that their people can routinely access. Make it as easy as possible by e-mailing employees your best site list—be sure to include the appropriate hot links.

TAKE ACTION!

Visit the Center for Science in the Public Interest's website at www.cspinet.org and check out the credible sites that they have identified—from private health organizations to government entities—this is a site you won't want to miss.

GREAT IDEA #37

Make the time. Work stoppage doesn't excite any employer, but consider the potential benefits of reduced health risks that won't result without strategic intervention at the worksite. Chevron Corporation employs an estimated 28,000 people.[39] Most of their programs are delivered on company time, resulting in extraordinary participation rates—exceeding 70%. A study conducted on this type of programming revealed that as participation increased, medical expenditures decreased. In addition, regular participants of the fitness centers experienced 54% fewer lost workdays than non-participants.[40]

TAKE ACTION!

Convene a "task force" of decision makers to explore the idea of creating a policy that allows employees regular amounts of time to participate in company sanctioned health and wellness events. To many, this may seem like a daunting task, but remember: Without these kinds of policies, it's hard to get mid-level managers and other key gatekeepers to really support wellness activities.

GREAT IDEA #38

Cake mistakes. We know that it's a nice thought, but a cake for every special occasion adds up. Try to monitor the food that's offered at company parties. This doesn't mean that you have to serve rice cakes and celery all the time, but try to keep a balance of the food that's offered. Instead of cake, why not serve frozen yogurt? This helps make the statement that your company is health conscious.

TAKE ACTION!

First you'll need to identify the special events—both formal and informal—where food is routinely provided. Where food is catered in, it will be important to work closely with those vendors to provide healthy alternatives. For those informal events where people bring food from home, it might be wise to create a cookbook of healthier recipes that people can access when it's their turn to provide the goodies.

The average American hand touches a refrigerator door 26 times a day. This number increases during the thirty days between Thanksgiving and Christmas when the average American gains six pounds of fat.[41]

**Robert Sweetgall,
Walk the Four Seasons
Walking and Cross-Training Log Book**

Great Idea #39

Be a role model. Make positive lifestyle changes and get involved in your programs. Employees value the image of senior executives. *The Journal of the American Medical Association* discusses the relationship between leadership and physical activity—most U.S. citizens value the healthy lifestyles of our nation's leaders. From the boxing and hunting of Teddy Roosevelt to the swimming of FDR, the touch football of John Kennedy and the jogging of Jimmy Carter.[18]

Take Action!

Identify and enroll a wellness champion within your organization to serve as chairperson of your event or campaign. Make sure to provide your employees with their bio and a laundry list of how that particular senior level executive stays healthy.

Great Idea #40

Size matters. Educate employees on portion sizes. According to clinical studies, Americans underestimate the amount of calories they consume each day by as much as 25%.[42] Display plates of food in the company cafeteria of proper portion sizes (i.e., 3 ounces of meat is about equal to the size of a cassette tape, and 3 ounces of fish is equal to the size if a checkbook). Also provide customized plates that have portion sizes printed on them.

Take Action!

For more information on the daily caloric recommendations and portion sizes, visit the American Dietetic Association at www.eatright.org.

The second-fastest-growing cable channel is the Food Network, whose audience grew in 1997 and reached into 27 million homes.[26]

"We can now prove that large numbers of Americans are dying from sitting on their behinds."

—Bruce B. Dan

GREAT IDEA #41

Analyze this. Encourage employees to have their family recipes analyzed by a dietician. This analysis can identify high-fat, high-caloric ingredients and perhaps recommend substitutions to make it a healthier meal.

TAKE ACTION!

**Create an event where employees can meet with
local dietitians and nutritionists to have their favorite
recipes analyzed and modified. Make sure to keep track
of all of the modified recipes and create a company cookbook that
contains dozens of great tasting and healthier recipes.
Oh by the way, your local health care provider,
county health department, or extension agent can help
you locate the right people—for free!**

GREAT IDEA #42

Showcase new toys. Each year, new fitness "toys" emerge in the marketplace. Not only are these toys fun, but many can also be extremely useful. Take, for example, DigiWalker™. This small device is actually a high tech pedometer that records a person's physical activity during the course of the day. Users can check their results online and even compare their activity levels against others who wear the device.

TAKE ACTION!

**To find out more about DigiWalker™ check out
www.digiwalker.com. Once you've learned more about this great
tool, negotiate a discount for your employees and then create contests
where employees are encouraged to take 10,000 steps a day.**

GREAT IDEA #43

efore and happily ever after. Some success stories are best conveyed by using visual aids as proof of an accomplishment. Good examples are before and after photographs or displaying old oversized pants that an individual used to wear before they lost weight. These are powerful proof-based illustrations that can help motivate those who are contemplating to lose weight, preparing for a weight loss program, trying to shed pounds, or fighting to maintain their new figure.

TAKE ACTION!

Search out these success stories at your organization and encourage successful individuals to share their experiences. Create a display of before and after clothing. Sound hoaky? Think about the testimonials that were provided by "case studies" of Subway restaurants—it was worth millions.

Approximately two-thirds of persons who lose weight will regain it within a year, and almost all persons who lose weight will regain it within five years.[43]

GREAT IDEA #44

ust say yes! Educate about pharmaceutical interventions. A review of 44 pharmacotherapy articles provides strong evidence that pharmacological therapy (which has generally been studied along with lifestyle modification, including diet, and physical activity) results in weight loss in obese adults when used six months to a year.[44] Advise your employees to see a physician to explore all of the possible options.

TAKE ACTION!

Learn more about pharmaceutical interventions as they relate to individual weight loss. We encourage you to visit www. rocheusa.com where you'll find more information about specific therapies for weight loss including new drugs like Xenical.

GREAT IDEA #45

eward with healthy incentives. Congratulations! Your program has been successful—employees have lost weight and they're keeping it off. So what do you reward them with? A double-decker chocolate cake? No, of course not. As incentives, give away cookbooks that focus on healthy nutritious recipes, such as the American Heart Association's *Low-Fat, Low-Cholesterol Cookbook* or the American Cancer Society's *Healthy Eating Cookbook*. Running shoes or other athletic gear is another fun and healthy reward.

TAKE ACTION!

Put together a brief brainstorming session to identify a laundry list of potential incentives that could be used within your organization. Make sure to include your most creative employees in this important meeting. Once you've created your list, carefully scrutinize each item for it's overall appeal and value—don't put this off.

> *"The biggest seller is cookbooks and the second is diet books—how not to eat what you've just learned how to cook."*
> —**Andy Rooney**

GREAT IDEA #46

Teach a cooking class. Not only has Offutt Air Force Base transformed the hangar that once housed the infamous Enola Gay into a world-class fitness center, it has also built a full kitchen for cooking demonstrations and nutrition classes. And, the kitchen comes complete with a consulting dietitian!

TAKE ACTION!

Offer a cooking demonstration over the lunch hour. To do this you'll need to identify talented "cooks" within your community who have the charisma to hold your employees' attention. Check with your local hospitals to begin your search. Think about the number of viewers that watch cooking channels—your employees are going to love this idea!

GREAT IDEA #47

Mark it off. Highsmith Inc. located in rural Fort Atkinson, WI, has a beautiful view of the surrounding countryside—and their metered walking trail reveals it. By marking exact distances, employees not only know how far they're walking, but they can also estimate the number of calories they've burned during their exercise break.

TAKE ACTION!

Identify the most traveled areas in and around your organization and measure the distances carefully. Once completed, format this information into a communiqué and circulate it to all employees. In addition, you may want to create "fitness" maps that outline specific routes that your employees can access. A great website that will give you some additional ideas is www.mapquest.com.

GREAT IDEA #48

W eigh in. Place scales throughout the organization. Scales raise consciousness about weight. And a raised consciousness can incite action. Although a bit unusual, having scales located throughout the organization sends a message. One caution: make sure that the scale's location provides a modest level of privacy so that people don't have to share their numbers with the world.

TAKE ACTION!

Here's a great way to get your organization involved
in a weight loss competition. Divide your employees into teams.
Collectively weigh each team on a large industrial scale—
if your organization doesn't have one, you can find them
at places like the Post Office or other organizations that
weigh large objects. After employees engage in exercise
and weight loss programs, you can weigh each team again
and measure the amount of weight lost. This provides
camaraderie and anonymity.

> *"Desperation is a fellow shaving before stepping on the scales."*
>
> **—Unknown**

GREAT IDEA #49

ighlight success stories. Create a "wall of fame" showcasing your company's healthiest employees. By showcasing employees who have successfully conquered the battle of the bulge, you not only reward individual accomplishments, but also encourage others at the same time.

TAKE ACTION!

Identify ten—count 'em ten—testimonials that can bring weight loss issues to the forefront. Be sure to make each person's story compelling and personal. These testimonials can be included in company newsletters, e-mails, and on bulletin boards. Even though employees may gain the weight back, it's important to emphasize the realities of behavior change—it lets other employees know that no one's perfect.

GREAT IDEA #50

tep up to the scale. Now it's your turn to weigh in. Do you know how your program fared? Was it a success? Can it be changed for the better? Don't expect perfection right away, but do strive for it over time. Consistently evaluating your program will allow you to recognize what's working and what's not.

TAKE ACTION!

Write down your definition of a successful weight loss program before it gets underway. After all is said and done, ask yourself if you were successful. Evaluating can be as easy as pre and post program weight measurement, simple surveys, and participation rates— but remember not everything that counts is countable. You'll want to make sure that you take employee feedback into account when measuring the success of your program.

> *"The toughest thing about being a success is that you've got to keep on being a success."*
>
> —**Irving Berlin**

> *"It is not only for what we do that we are held responsible, but also for what we do not do."*
>
> —**Moliere**

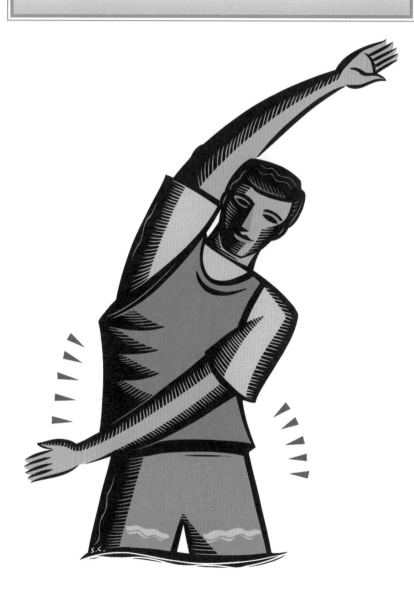

LOOKING AHEAD

Now's the hard part. It's time for you to take these ideas from the pages, determine your intentions, and translate those intentions into reality. It won't be easy—successful health promotion programming is just as much art as it is science. It takes creativity and hard work. You'll need to carefully collect data, tailor your initiatives to your specific population, and carry out routine evaluations if you want your programs to make an impact at the workplace.

To help you get started, we've included a checklist on the following pages. You will find a series of questions that address the various components of results-oriented wellness programs—everything from senior level support to evaluation strategies.

Above all, do something! It's likely that not every idea in this book will align with your specific wellness efforts. Nevertheless, the driving message behind each idea is to stimulate creative thinking and get you to take action. And remember, you don't need to change the world today—even small changes throughout the workplace can lead to big improvements.

THE WELL WORKPLACE CHECKLIST

Contrary to popular belief, there's more to worksite wellness than building fitness centers and conducting brown bag seminars. For over ten years, we at the Wellness Councils of America have been helping organizations of all kinds to develop and deliver world-class wellness programs—the kind of initiatives that change organizational culture and transform lives.

If there is one thing we have learned over the course of our existence, it's this; success doesn't just happen by accident. Indeed, in order to create the kind of results that count—healthier employees and a more competitive organization—a wellness program must be carefully designed and flawlessly executed.

So how do you know if your program is on the right track? That's where the "Well Workplace Checklist" comes in.

We encourage you to answer all of the questions as honestly and accurately as you can. Remember, this checklist is simply a tool that is designed to help you see if your wellness program is on the right track—there are no right or wrong answers. So relax, take a deep breath and get started.

I. Senior Level Support

Support for our organization's wellness initiative is demonstrated by the fact that:
(please check appropriate response)

1. Our CEO genuinely believes in the value of worksite wellness. ☐ Yes ☐ No

2. A statement concerning employee health and well-being has been incorporated into the company's vision/mission statement. ☐ Yes ☐ No

3. Our CEO has communicated the importance of wellness to all employees (e.g., formal written memo, incorporated into orientation, public addresses, etc.). ☐ Yes ☐ No

4. The company has formally appointed an individual(s) and/or a committee to lead the wellness initiative. ☐ Yes ☐ No

5. Senior level management allocates the necessary resources for the wellness program (e.g., budget, materials, people, space, etc.). ☐ Yes ☐ No

Senior Level Support (cont.)

6. Our CEO and senior level executives regularly take part in the activities offered.   ☐ Yes ☐ No

7. Middle level management supports the wellness initiative for the organization's employees (e.g., provide time to participate, actively promote wellness activities, etc.).   ☐ Yes ☐ No

8. Middle level management regularly participates in wellness activities.   ☐ Yes ☐ No

II. The Wellness Team

Integration of the health promotion program is demonstrated by the fact that: (please check the appropriate response)

1. A representative wellness committee involving the organizations' key employees/constituents has been established (e.g., human resource/benefits, occupational health, MIS, etc.).   ☐ Yes ☐ No

2. The wellness committee has developed a compelling vision, established strategic priorities, and defined individual roles and responsibilities.   ☐ Yes ☐ No

3. The wellness committee has a strong and effective leader.   ☐ Yes ☐ No

4. The wellness committee functions cohesively and effectively.   ☐ Yes ☐ No

5. The wellness committee meets regularly throughout the year.   ☐ Yes ☐ No

6. The proceedings of the meetings are consistently communicated to senior level executives.   ☐ Yes ☐ No

III. Data Collection

In order to make strategic decisions, the following sources of data have been collected and analyzed within the last: (please check the appropriate response)

	Months				Have not collected
	12	24	36	48	
Health risk appraisals	☐	☐	☐	☐	☐
Health screening (e.g., height, weight, blood profile, etc.)	☐	☐	☐	☐	☐
Employee health interest surveys	☐	☐	☐	☐	☐
Health needs/interests of dependents and/or retirees	☐	☐	☐	☐	☐
Physical fitness assessments	☐	☐	☐	☐	☐
Work/family needs assessment	☐	☐	☐	☐	☐
Ergonomic/work station analysis	☐	☐	☐	☐	☐

	Months				Have not
	12	24	36	48	collected
Facility assessment	❏	❏	❏	❏	❏
Demographic information of employees/dependents	❏	❏	❏	❏	❏
Health care claims and utilization	❏	❏	❏	❏	❏
Absenteeism records	❏	❏	❏	❏	❏
Disability claims	❏	❏	❏	❏	❏
Worker compensation claims	❏	❏	❏	❏	❏
Injury records	❏	❏	❏	❏	❏
Corporate culture audit	❏	❏	❏	❏	❏
Union support	❏	❏	❏	❏	❏
Policy assessment	❏	❏	❏	❏	❏

IV. Annual Operating Plan

In order to provide clarity and focus to our wellness initiative, we have: (please check the appropriate response)

1. Carefully developed an operating plan that addresses our employees' health needs and interests. ❏ Yes ❏ No

2. Established clear, concise, and measurable goals and objectives that are linked to and supported by data. ❏ Yes ❏ No

3. Linked our wellness goals and objectives to the organization's strategic priorities and outcomes. ❏ Yes ❏ No

4. Incorporated specific timelines within the operating plan indicating when activities/tasks are to be completed. ❏ Yes ❏ No

5. Assigned specific responsibilities to an individual or group for the completion of important tasks. ❏ Yes ❏ No

6. Allocated an itemized budget sufficient to carry out the plan. ❏ Yes ❏ No

7. Incorporated appropriate marketing strategies to effectively promote and communicate our programs to the employees and their dependents. ❏ Yes ❏ No

8. A plan to evaluate the stated goals and objectives. ❏ Yes ❏ No

V. Programs and Interventions

To address the health needs and interests of our employees and their dependents, our organization has offered the following programs in the last 24 months: (please check all that apply)

	Program Formats:				
	Health Information	Group Education	Self Study	Computer Based	Personal Counseling
Physical activity	❑	❑	❑	❑	❑
Smoking cessation	❑	❑	❑	❑	❑
Nutrition/weight management	❑	❑	❑	❑	❑
Responsible alcohol use	❑	❑	❑	❑	❑
Stress management	❑	❑	❑	❑	❑
Medical self-care	❑	❑	❑	❑	❑
Work and family	❑	❑	❑	❑	❑
Personal financial management	❑	❑	❑	❑	❑
Safety/health protection	❑	❑	❑	❑	❑
Ergonomics	❑	❑	❑	❑	❑
Mental health/depression	❑	❑	❑	❑	❑
Disease management (e.g., asthma, diabetes, etc.)	❑	❑	❑	❑	❑
Other	❑	❑	❑	❑	❑

Are any of the above programs:

offered to employees' families?   ❑ Yes ❑ No

offered to retirees?   ❑ Yes ❑ No

Does the organization regularly participate in community health promotion or social service activities (i.e., blood drives, run/walk-a-thon, clothing/food drives)?   ❑ Yes ❑ No

VI. Supportive Environments

In order to provide a supportive organizational environment, we: (please check the appropriate response)

1. Provide our employees with release time so that they can participate in our health promotion activities. ☐ Yes ☐ No

2. Practice disability prevention and management (e.g., early return to work, restricted duty, etc.). ☐ Yes ☐ No

3. Reimburse our employees for health club memberships and/or other wellness programs. ☐ Yes ☐ No

4. Provide incentives to our employees to increase participation in our wellness initiatives. ☐ Yes ☐ No

5. Offer our employees peer support groups and mentoring opportunities. ☐ Yes ☐ No

6. Make healthy food options available in our vending machines and cafeteria. ☐ Yes ☐ No

7. Ensure that all workstations are ergonomically sound. ☐ Yes ☐ No

8. Monitor our facility's heating, lighting, ventilation, and overall safety. ☐ Yes ☐ No

9. Maintain an easily accessible wellness library. ☐ Yes ☐ No

10. Offer assistance to help employees address issues of work/life balance. ☐ Yes ☐ No

11. Recognize and reward successes. ☐ Yes ☐ No

12. Provide the following benefit options (check all that apply):

☐ Health insurance
☐ Dependent care flexible spending accounts
☐ Disability
☐ Health promotion program prepayment or reimbursement
☐ Life insurance
☐ Sick leave/well days off
☐ Leave of absence
☐ Compensatory time off
☐ Vacation

☐ Flex time
☐ Job sharing
☐ Work at home/telecommuting
☐ Maternal/paternal leave
☐ Family leave
☐ Child care
☐ Retirement/investment plan
☐ Tuition reimbursement
☐ EAP
☐ Others (please list) _____

Supportive Environments (cont.)

13. In order to provide a supportive organizational environment, we provide the following policies (check all that apply):

❏ Smoke free workplace
❏ Tobacco restrictions
❏ Seatbelt/safe driving practices
❏ Alcohol/drugs
❏ Healthy food options
❏ Emergency procedures
❏ Other (please list) _____

VII. Evaluation

Our organization is committed to evaluating our wellness program in the following ways: (please check the appropriate response)

1. Regularly tracking participation. ❏ Yes ❏ No

2. Monitoring participant satisfaction. ❏ Yes ❏ No

3. Documenting improvements in knowledge, attitudes, skills, and behaviors. ❏ Yes ❏ No

4. Assessing changes in biometric measures (e.g., body weight, strength, flexibility, cholesterol levels, blood pressure, etc.). ❏ Yes ❏ No

5. Assessing and monitoring the health status of "at-risk" employees. ❏ Yes ❏ No

6. Measuring changes in both the physical and cultural environment (e.g., policies, benefits, working conditions, etc.). ❏ Yes ❏ No

7. Monitoring the impact of wellness on key productivity indicators (e.g., absenteeism, turnover, morale, etc.). ❏ Yes ❏ No

8. Analyzing cost effectiveness, cost savings, and return on investment. ❏ Yes ❏ No

VIII. Communication

To keep all members of the organization informed, we regularly and continuously: (please check the appropriate response)

1. Provide program updates to senior level executives. ❏ Yes ❏ No

2. Circulate information concerning the availability of community resources (e.g., child care, elder care, parks, etc.). ❏ Yes ❏ No

3. Communicate changes in policy and benefit options. ❏ Yes ❏ No

4. Distribute reminders to employees and their families concerning upcoming activities and events. ❏ Yes ❏ No

5. Encourage ongoing dialogue by providing opportunities for employee input. ❏ Yes ❏ No

6. Provide timely feedback to individuals that are involved in the company's programs. ❏ Yes ❏ No

7. Allow employees to communicate feedback through formal communication channels (e.g., suggestion boxes, e-mail, surveys, etc.). ❏ Yes ❏ No

8. Communicate program results to all levels of management. ❏ Yes ❏ No

REFERENCES

[1] National Vital Statistics Report, Vol. 48 No. 11.

[2] McGinnis, J. Michael & Foege, William H. *Actual Causes of Death in the United States.* Journal of the American Medical Association. November 10, 1993. Vol. 270, No. 18. pg. 2208.

[3] Thompson, et al. 1998. *Estimated Economic Costs of Obesity to U.S. Business.* The American Journal of Health Promotion, Vol. 13, No. 2.

[4] Business & Health Special Report. *Weighty Matters: Obesity, Health and Productivity.* August, 1998. Vol. 16, No. 8, Supplement A.

[5] Nestle, Marion and Jacobson, Michael. *Halting the Obesity Epidemic: A Public Health Policy Approach.* Public Health Reports. January/February 2000. Vol. 115 pg. 18.

[6] Burton, WB, et.al. *The Economic Costs Associated with Body Mass Index in a Workplace.* Journal of Occupational and Environmental Medicine. 1998, Vol. 40 No. 9 pp. 786-792.

[7] Caan, B, et al. *Increases in Pharmacy Costs Among Obese Members in an HMO* [abstract]. Obesity Research 1999. Vol. 7 (suppl 1) 54S. Abstract O146.

[8] The Wellness Councils of America. *Healthy Wealthy & Wise: Fundamentals of Workplace Health Promotion.* P.24, 1995.

[9] *The Health Project: C. Everett Koop National Health Award Winners.* healthproject.Stanford.edu/koop/Caterpillar/description.html and healthproject.stanford.edu/koop/Caterpillar/evaluation.html.

[10] Serdula, M., et al. *Prevalence of Attempting Weight Loss and Strategies for Controlling Weight.* The Journal of the American Medical Association. Vol.282, No.14, 1999, pp.1353-1358.

[11] Good Housekeeping. *Bye-Bye Belly?* http://goodhousekeeping.women.com/gh/diet/fitness/27bell11.htm.

[12] Federal Trade Commission. *Diet Workshop to Settle FTC Charges Weight Loss Claims Were Deceptive.* http://www.ftc.gov/opa/1996/9603/diet.htm. March 1996.

[13] Federal Trade Commission. *FTC Announces "Operation Waistline" –A Law Enforcement and Consumer Education Effort Designed to Stop Misleading Weight Loss Claims.* http://www.ftc.gov/opa/1997/9703/waistlin.htm. March 1997.

[14] Borushek, Allan. *The Doctor's Pocket Calorie Fat Counter.* Family Health Publications, 1997.

[15] MSNBC. *Vending Machines go High-Tech.* http://stacks.msnbc.com/news/552126.asp.

[16] Centers for Disease Control and Prevention. *Physical Activity and Good Nutrition: Essential Elements for Good Health.* Pg. 3.

[17] U.S. Department of Health and Human Services. *Physical Activity and Health: A Report of the Surgeon General.* Atlanta, GA: U.S. Department of Health and Human Services, Centers for Disease Control and Prevention and Health Promotion, 1996.

[18] Koplan, Jeffrey P. and Dietz, William H. *Caloric Imbalance and Public Health Policy.* The Journal of the American Medical Association. Vol. 282 No. 16.

[19] Centers for Disease Control and Prevention's (CDC) National Health and Nutrition Examination Survey (NHANES). *Prevalence of Overweight Among Children and Adolescents: United States, 1999.* www.cdc.gov/nchs/products/pubs/pubd/hestats/over99fig1.htm.

[20] *The World Almanac and Book of Facts.* World Almanac Education Group 2001.

[21] Krantz, Les. *America by the Numbers: Facts and Figures from the Weighty to the Way-Out.* Houghton Mifflin Company. 1993. p. 206.

[22] Tate, Deborah F., et al. *Using Internet Technology to Deliver a Behavioral Weight Loss Program.* The Journal of the American Medical Association. Vol. 285, No. 9.

[23] Letterman, D., et al. *David Letterman's Book of Top Ten Lists and Zesty Lo-Cal Chicken Recipes.* Bantam Books, 1995.

[24] The National Soft Drink Association. *About Soft Drinks.* www.nsda.org/softdrinks/history/funfacts.html.

[25] Marcus, Bess H., and Forsyth, LeighAnn H. *How Are We Doing With Physical Activity?* American Journal of Health Promotion. Vol 14, No. 2.

[26] Naisbitt, John. *High Tech High Touch.* Broadway Books, 1999.

[27] National Restaurant Association. *Industry at a Glance.* www.restaurant.org/research/ind_glance.html.

[28] Schlosser, Eric. *Fast Food Nation, The Dark Side of the All-American Meal.* Houghton Mifflin Company, 2001.

[29] *Reader's Digest Book of Facts. Marvels of the Human Body.* Reader's Digest Association, 1995.

[30] Kassirer, J.P. and Angell, M. *Losing Weight—An Ill-Fated New Year's Resolution.* The New England Journal of Medicine. Vol. 338 No. 1.

[31] Lamberg, Lynne. *Psychiatric Help May Shrink Some Waistlines.* The Journal of the American Medical Association. Vol. 284. No. 3.

[32] Weigh To Health, Fat Gram Indicator, Roche Pharmaceuticals.

[33] Willet, Walter, C et al. *Guidelines for Healthy Weight.* The New England Journal of Medicine. Vol. 341. No. 6.

[34] NHLBI. *Clinical Guidelines on the Identification, Evaluation, and Treatment of Overweight and Obesity in Adults—Executive Summary.* Clinical Guidelines. www.nhlbi.nih.gov/guidelines/obesity/sum_clin.htm.

[35] Fontanarosa, Phil B. *Patients, Physicians, and Weight Control.* The Journal of the American Medical Association. Volume 282. No. 16.

[36] *McDonald's USA Nutrition Facts.* www.mcdonalds.com/countries/usa/food/nutrition_facts/sandfries/sandfries.html.

[37] About Crisco. Product Information. www.crisco.com/prod_info.htm.

[38] *The World Almanac and Book of Facts 2000.* Primedia Reference, Inc., 2000.

[39] Chevron Profile. Chevron Today. www.chevron.com/about/overview/profile.shtml.

[40] The Health Project: C. Everett Koop National Health Award Winners. healthproject.Stanford.edu/koop/Chevron/description.html and healthproject.stanford.edu/koop/Chevron/evaluation.html.

[41] Sweetgall, Robert. *Walk the Four Seasons: Walking and Cross-Training Log Book.* Creative Walking Inc. 1992.

[42] American Institute for Cancer Research. *Nutritionists Warn Public: Portion Sizes Out of Control.* http://www.aicr.org/r102099.htm.

[43] Rosenbaum, Michael. *Review Article: Medical Progress. Obesity.* The New England Journal of Medicine.

[44] NHLBI. *Clinical Guidelines on the Identification, Evaluation, and Treatment of Overweight and Obesity in Adults—Executive Summary.* Summary of Evidence-Based Recommendations. www.nhlbi.nih.gov/guidelines/obesity/sum_rec.htm.

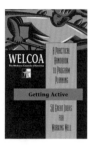
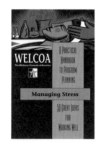
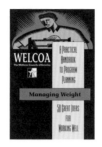
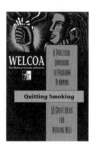
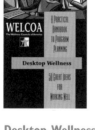
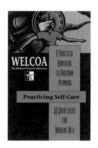

About the Authors

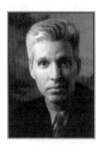

Our Editors

David Hunnicutt, PhD is the President of the Wellness Councils of America (WELCOA). Under his leadership and direction WELCOA has become a leader in the production of organizational and consumer health information. Widely published, David speaks frequently on the topics of corporate wellness, effective leadership, and healthy job design. He is currently working on his second book titled *The Competitive Advantage of Healthy Companies.*

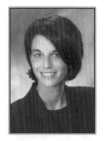

Brittanie Leffelman is the assistant to the President and manages major writing projects at WELCOA. With a Master's Degree in Health Promotion, Brittanie has coordinated national health forums, major grants, and state and local wellness initiatives.

WELCOA Writing Staff

The WELCOA writing staff is responsible for the development of a vast array of leading-edge health publications. Over the last several years WELCOA writers have produced a monthly health and wellness newsletter that has a circulation that reaches more than three million employees each year. In addition, our writers have recently completed *Self-Care Essentials: A Simple Guide to Managing Your Health Care and Living Well*—a self-care book that will be disseminated to hundreds of thousands of employees this year alone.

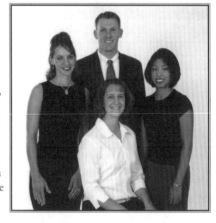

- **Craig Johnson** is the Managing Editor for WELCOA. He received his B.S. in Exercise Science from Nebraska Wesleyan University in Lincoln, Nebraska in 1999. He is currently pursuing an M.A. in Health and Wellness Management.
- **Carie Maguire** (left) is a Staff Writer who received her B.A. in Journalism with an emphasis in Public Relations from the University of Nebraska at Omaha.
- **Sara Spurgin** (center) is a Staff Writer who received her B.F.A. in Creative Writing from the University of Nebraska at Omaha.
- **Marice Reyes** (right) is a Staff Writer who earned her B.S. in Exercise Science from Creighton University in Omaha, Nebraska.

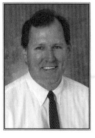

Our Designer

David Trouba, WELCOA's Creative Director, oversees the design of all materials produced by WELCOA. His acumen for creating engaging publications is demonstrated through the materials he has produced—including national health communications kits, calendars, numerous marketing pieces, and website graphic development. David has over two decades of experience in graphic design, and comes to WELCOA after a 10-year career at Hallmark Cards, Inc. in Kansas City, MO.